ALL THINGS GIRL

Mirror, Mirror, on the Wall... What is Beauty After All?

**TERESA TOMEO
MOLLY MILLER
MONICA COPS**

© 2008 by Teresa Tomeo, Molly Miller, and Monica Cops

The "All Things Girl" series is published by
Bezalel Books
Waterford, MI
www.BezalelBooks.com

All titles in the ALL THINGS GIRL series:
Friends, Boys, and Getting Along
Mirror, Mirror on the Wall…What is Beauty After All?
Girls Rock!
Mind Your Manners
Modern and Modest
All Things Girl Journal

Printed in the United States of America. All rights reserved. No part of this publication may be reproduced, stored in a retrieval system, or transmitted in any form or by any means-for example, electronic, photocopy, recording-without the prior written permission of the author. The only exception is brief quotations in printed reviews.

Authors' note: This book is intended to be used as a tool for parents of "tween" Catholic girls. It broaches many subjects that are personal in nature and is written with the belief and understanding that the primary educator of children is the parents. This book gently threads the truths of many of JPII's teachings throughout while addressing the real issues and physical changes that take place in young girls. While not all the titles in this series address such personal matters, "Mirror, Mirror" does so in such a way as to provide every young girl with information meant to be used in conversations that take place in the privacy and love of the Catholic home.

References to the Catechism of the Catholic Church are denoted: CCC

ISBN 978-0-9818854-2-1
Library of Congress Control Number 2008931734

THIS BOOK IS DEDICATED TO...

To my mom, Rose,
Thank you for all of your sacrifices and especially thank you for the gift of life.
Teresa

To my mom, Maureen,
Thank you for always telling me I was beautiful. I love you, mom.
Your loving daughter, Molly

To my mom, Maricruz,
Thank you for teaching me what True Beauty is all about; and to Our Lady, Mother Most Beautiful.
Monica

Contents

High Class ... 5

Princess ... 7

Take it From Teresa ... 9

Stages and Changes ... 13

Make These Yourself ... 21

Basic Skincare ... 23

Hair ... 27

Nails ... 35

Virtues to Live By ... 40

Have a Plan! ... 46

A Girl Like Me ... 49

High Class

All people begin life in their mother's womb. From the beginning of your creation, tiny as you were, you were a person. Being created a person, and not, let's say, a kitty or a dog, is special because God gave you a soul that will live forever. A person is a creature made up of a body and a soul. As a person, you are in a "higher class" because your soul is what gives you "the image and likeness of God". Your Creator, God the Father has stamped on your soul, dignity. What is dignity? It is your worth as a person.

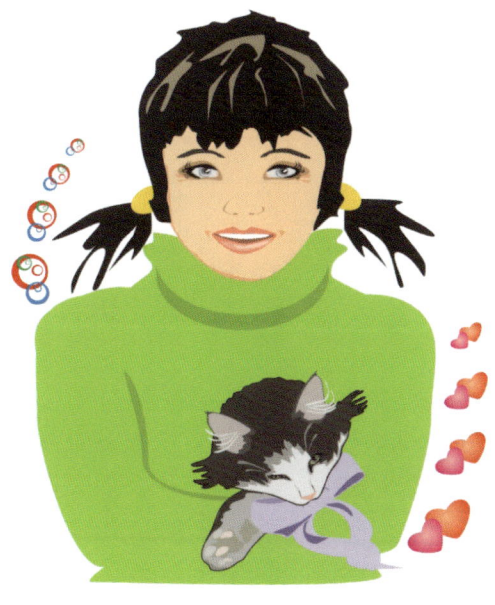

Dignity has three characteristics:

1) You have it no matter what circumstances you live in.
2) You have it no matter what you look like.
3) You have it, no matter what changes you go through in your life.

Here are some examples of dignity...

Jennifer lives in a neighborhood where the houses are very small and the people work hard but don't have much money. Katie lives in a mansion and takes expensive vacations every year. *Which person has more dignity?*

Jade is from Africa and has deep brown skin. Julie has red hair and freckles. Laura is chubby. Maggie is tall and skinny. *Which girl has more dignity?*

Opal is 95 years old and lives in a nursing home and has to be spoon fed. Riley was in a car accident and has a huge scar on her face. Jessica is a beautiful movie star. *Which person has more dignity?*

Hopefully you answered "neither" to all of the examples because all people are equal in dignity. You will go through good and bad times, happiness and sadness, success and failure in your life. Sometimes people think these things are what define you. This is a lie you must not believe.

At this point you should be feeling pretty good about yourself.

Just in case you need more, check it out, it gets better!

Always remember that your dignity is a precious gift from God!

Princess

When you were a baby, your mom and dad brought you to church to be baptized. What does baptism do? It washes away original sin, makes you a child of God and fills your soul with grace. God is the King of the universe, and you are His daughter: that makes you a princess! As a princess in the royal family of God, you have a value greater than a rare jewel and He loves you soooooo much. This is what defines you as a person and nothing, including popularity, good grades, designer clothes or money, makes a difference in who you are in the sight of God your Father.

So you see, you are so much more than body parts. You are intelligent, creative and caring. You are not an object, but a person, and a female person at that! Sexuality is what makes you a girl, different from males. Only a woman can carry another living person within her body. God also gave to women unique gifts such as a nurturing heart, a giving spirit, and a detail oriented mind. These gifts are used for the good of those around you and for your own true happiness.

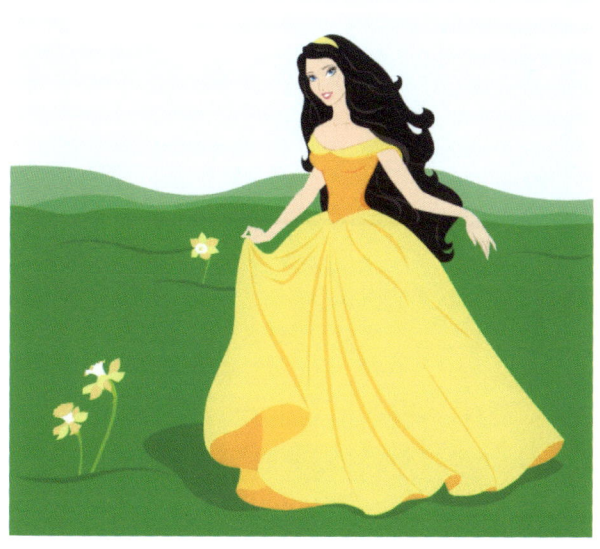

Lots of girls grow up trying to answer the soul searching question of *"Why am I here?"*

The answer is simple; *To know, love, and serve God in this life and to be happy with Him forever in Heaven in the next.*

You get to *know, love and serve God from Jesus Christ, the Son of God, who teaches us through the Catholic Church.*

But how do you do all these? Let's go step by step:

1. To know God:

What would you do if you want to get to know a movie star? You'd try to read up all the information about him or her in magazines and books, you would watch interviews on T.V., ask people around you what they know, etc. Well, you get to know God in a similar way: reading the Bible, listening to your parents talk about God, listening in religion class seriously, praying and receiving the Sacraments.

2. To love God:

Did you ever notice that when you have a really good friend you want to spend more and more time with her? And then, the more time you spend with her the more you love her? It's the same way with God. To love God, you need to spend time with Him in prayer, adoring and thanking Him for your blessings, and worshipping Him at Sunday Mass. The amazing thing is, just like with a good friend, the more time you spend with God the more you will love Him!

3. To Serve God:

You serve God by serving other people. Serving God is doing daily chores cheerfully without complaining. You serve God when you serve other people through your kind words and compassionate ways. You serve God when you participate in community service projects or do things like visit residents in a nursing home. God is in each and every person so when you serve other people, you are serving God!

*As you grow up,
ask Our Lord in what special way
He wants you to know, love and serve Him.
This will be your vocation
and will make you truly happy in your life.*

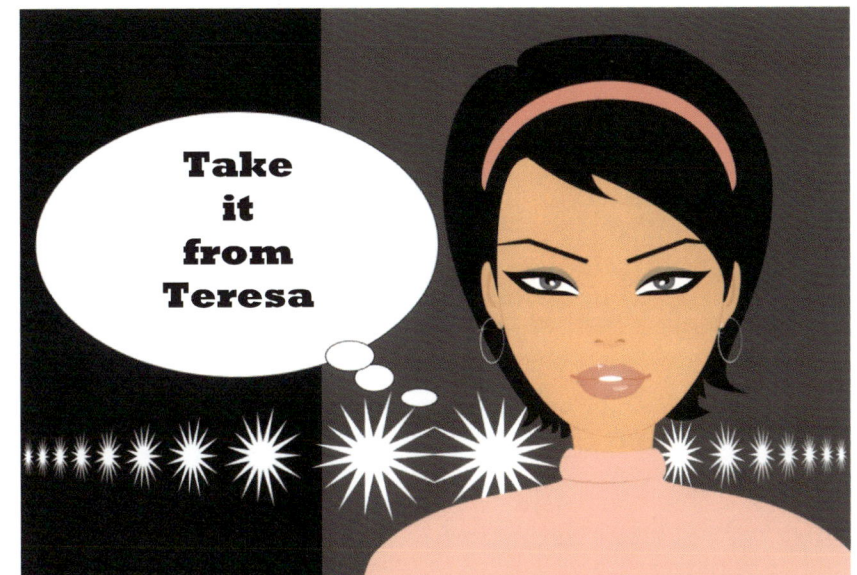

Let me ask you a very important question...

What do you see when you look in the mirror?

Hopefully, no matter what your size or shape, no matter the color of your skin, hair, or eyes, when you look in the mirror you see what the Lord sees; a princess and a beautiful daughter of God. Take it from me, as someone who works in the media, and someone who has been greatly impacted by the culture, which puts constant pressure on ladies of all ages to look or dress a certain way, I know that it is hard not to compare yourself to a cover girl or your favorite TV star. We are all bombarded with messages 24/7 from the Internet, television, music videos, billboards, magazine covers, and more. So to say that none of us is going to be impacted by the mass media is like saying we can walk outside in a rainstorm without our umbrella and not get wet.

Did you know that even Chinese officials recently felt pressure from the world's mistaken concept of external beauty? At the last minute, as they were getting ready for the opening ceremonies of the Summer Olympics that would be broadcast around the world to millions and millions of viewers, these officials decided to replace a young singer with a Chinese child star whom they deemed to be "prettier" than the 7 year old vocalist. The actress, who is apparently well known to Chinese TV viewers through numerous television commercials, was used to lip-synch a Chinese ballad over the other little girl's voice. Thank goodness Chinese officials were strongly criticized for their image obsession; but, unfortunately this is a glaring example of what's happening in our world today with too much emphasis put on perfection of outward appearance. In the Old Testament, 1st Samuel 16:7 we read: "Man looks at the outward appearance but God looks at the heart."

We are all impacted by what we see, hear, and read. But maybe after learning more about my particular challenges with media influence as a young girl, and maybe after seeing just how much time, effort, and money the mass media puts into trying to get your attention and your allowance money, you will think twice when you look in that mirror. Remember, always, no matter what, that you are a daughter of the King of Kings and the Lord of Lords and are always beautiful in His sight!

When I was growing up I always struggled with my weight. When I was about 12 years old I became more self conscious of my appearance and talked to my Mom about going on a diet. Mom took me to the pediatrician and they both agreed that losing a few pounds, maybe no more than 10 pounds or so, would be a good idea for my health. The doctor put me on a healthy well-balanced diet with lots of fruits and vegetables and I lost the weight fairly quickly. I looked good but for some reason, not good enough. I was secretly hoping that when I lost the weight I would be as thin as one of my idols on a Friday night TV show.

One of my favorite programs back when I was a tween in the early 70's was a situation comedy entitled, *"The Partridge Family,"* which revolved around a family of musicians who were performers that sang all over the country and traveled in their colorful tour bus. The characters on the show seemed to have so much fun and live such a glamorous life. They met so many interesting people and had the cutest matching outfits for their concerts! When I was growing up every young girl wanted to be a Partridge. One of the stars of the show was a beautiful young actress with long gorgeous hair. This actress was the "it girl" of my era and also a magazine cover girl. I had the long dark hair and convinced myself that if I could just lose a little more weight, I would look like my role model and my life would be perfect.

Well, a little more weight turned into losing more and more weight and before me or my family knew what had hit us, I had dieted myself down to a very dangerous 89 pounds. My Mom took me back to the pediatrician and the pediatrician marched me right off to the hospital so I could be monitored with the expectation of gaining some of my weight back.

My physician knew my desire to be thin wasn't normal but she didn't know much about my condition. Unfortunately, neither did the doctors at the hospital as eating disorders were just starting to get diagnosed back then.

However, by the end of my two-plus-weeks stay in the local children's hospital, I was finally diagnosed as having an eating disorder known as anorexia nervosa, an illness with which many people are now familiar. Consider all the coverage on the topic of celebrities being plagued by eating disorders including TV star Mary Kate Olsen of the famous Olsen twins, who was treated a few years ago for her battle with anorexia.

Since little was known about my disorder back then, there wasn't much the doctors could do except monitor my eating habits. When I started to gain a little weight they sent me home and I eventually moved on to high school. But I still suffer side effects today, more than three decades later.

According to ANRED, the Anorexia Nervosa and Related Eating Disorders organization (www.anred.com), anorexia is described as someone with a, *"relentless pursuit of thinness."* The organization also explains that a *"person suffering from anorexia also struggles to maintain a normal body weight, denies the dangers of their thinness, and is terrified of gaining weight even though she is alarmingly underweight."* Anorexia also might be rearing its ugly head if a person finds him or herself believing they are fat when they are actually thin or extremely thin. Anorexia is only one type of eating disorder but one of the common connections with eating disorder victims, and as you already know from my own reflections on my bout with anorexia, is media influence. Sadly, this is a major battle for all of us with the onslaught of messages coming at us that tell us we are only good enough if we are a certain size. Did you know that one lovely TV actress who is actually a size two was labeled as overweight by Hollywood reporters, and all because of one photo that was a bit unflattering?

Ladies, again, take it from me as a media insider and a survivor of anorexia, the devil uses the media to impact your self esteem and to take your mind off of the most important relationship in your life; your relationship with Jesus Christ and His Church. We are told that we are to love the Lord God with all our heart, mind, and strength. And how can we love God, or concentrate on growing in our relationship with Him, when we allow the media messages to tell us we are not lovable because we are not pretty or thin enough?

Please, don't do what I did and buy into all the media pressure! You may not see it as pressure, but it is! And, boy, is there a lot of it our there. How much?

Well for example, did you know that:

- *The average age for a girl to starting dieting is around your age – 8 years old.*
- *One out of every four TV commercials you see includes a message about appearance.*
- *81% of ten year olds in this country say they are afraid of being fat.*
- *One out of every three women is on a diet at any given time.*
- *Music videos featuring thin women can lead to an increase in your body dissatisfaction.*

If you can identify with any of the items in the list I just provided then it might be time to talk to Mom and Dad about your feelings. It is very important to address these issues early on. That way you can prevent a full-fledged eating disorder. Don't be ashamed. Your family loves you and God loves you and they want you to be the best you can be, and that means being free from the trap of low self esteem or an eating disorder.

Remember that the pull of the world is very strong. And again I am speaking from experience. If I can be greatly impacted years ago by just one TV show, how much stronger is the pull today with everything being thrown at you through the numerous media avenues?

When I was growing up we didn't have video games. We didn't have cable. We didn't have text messaging or cell phones. There were no Internet chat rooms or social gathering sites on the web and yet I still fell victim to the strong influences of the media. Most young people your age may not be aware of the media saturation because it is such a natural part of your environment. When you wake up in the morning you might turn on the radio or the TV and then head downstairs and start checking your e-mail before heading off to school. Many girls your age may have already owned at least one, if not several, cell phones or even lap tops. And then you're off to school and the media exposure starts all over again with friends texting each other between classes or on the bus ride. When you sit down to work on the computer you continue to be inundated with messages that really do impact you. And even if you don't see it yourself, your friends keep you "in the loop" about what is happening. I am sure that sometimes your heads must be spinning in trying to sort it all out.

It's also important to understand that advertisers, magazines, the TV networks, the department stores, and shopping malls don't exactly have your best interest in mind. They have your money or your parent's money in mind. How do I know this? I worked in the mainstream media for a very long time. Your age group, the 8 to 12 years olds or "tweens", represent a big dollar sign for advertisers, the music industry, clothing stores, designers, and cosmetic companies. Just how much money does that big dollar sign represent? How about 500 billion dollars a year? That's right. I said 500 billion dollars a year. That's a lot of money. And while there is nothing wrong with having nice things, the media wants you to think that you can't live without the latest Hannah Montana or Jonas Brothers t-shirt.

It's not that you can't enjoy certain elements of the media such as appropriate music or suitable TV shows. Don't get me wrong! I know that is a fun part of being your age, but in addition to obsession with appearance, there's also the pressure to buy more and more things. Things don't make you happy. That's what I'm trying to warn you against. God is the only one who can truly make you happy. Jesus tells us in Matthew 6:19-21 that we are not to "store up treasures on earth where moth and rust destroy and where thieves break in and steal." Instead we are to store up for ourselves "treasures in heaven, where moth and rust do not destroy, and where thieves do not break in and steal. For where your treasure is, there your heart will be also." The late great Pope John Paul II often said we don't find ourselves until we lose ourselves in Christ.

An eating disorder at the young age of 12 caused me to "store up" all my treasures in my appearance and my obsession to be skinny. That's all I thought about night and day. My heart was filled with vain thoughts and I was constantly worried about what I was eating and what I looked like and I was continually running from the bathroom scale to the bedroom mirror. That's not a healthy or a happy way to live. Possessions can do the same thing to us. But all those "earthly" things can be taken away from us very quickly. I did not want to be whisked off by my doctor to the local hospital, but there I was at 12 years old spending the first part of my summer in a hospital room missing out on all the fun because of my dangerous addiction to dieting.

Staying close to God and family is the best way to have a happy and healthy life. Have you ever heard of the saying "garbage in garbage out?" Well one of the important ways to help you stay on a positive path toward heaven is to apply balance and moderation and avoid the garbage or bad stuff. We've already talked about the garbage out there on the radio, TV, and the Internet so team up with Mom and Dad and let them know what programs and music you like. Ask them to discuss the shows with you to see if the CD's or TV shows match up to the morals that your parents are working so hard to instill in you and your brothers and sisters. Make sure you are following your parents' guidelines and don't spend too much time in front of the TV or computer. Go to the video store with Mom or Dad for a family movie night. Maybe pick out a movie about the life of your favorite young saint such as St. Claire of Assisi or St. Therese.

A few years ago there was a popular question that was showing up on jewelry, posters, coffee mugs, and just about everywhere else; What Would Jesus Do? Sometimes you would just see the initials "WWJD." Well I would like you to think about another question with similar initials. How about "WWJW," or, What Would Jesus Watch? Use these initials as a reminder and ask yourself that question before going to a certain website or watching a particular TV show. The question, along with the Holy Spirit, will help you and your family make healthy media choices.

And finally take the advice of someone else who loves you very much and prays for you every day: Pope Benedict XVI. Now, while the Pope may not know you by name, part of his responsibility as the successor of our first pope, St Peter, is to pray for the universal Church and all of her members including *you!* Maybe you sat down in school or at home to watch some of the coverage of his visit to the United States in April of 2008. He spent a lot of time with young people during his stops in the New York area and he told them to make time for God and not to be afraid of the silence.

"Have we perhaps lost something of the art of listening? Do you leave space to hear God's whisper, calling you forth into goodness? Friends, do not be afraid of silence or stillness, listen to God, and adore him in the Eucharist. Let his word shape your journey as an unfolding of holiness."

While it might be hard to find silence these days because of all of the daily noise in your life, take time to sit in silence with Jesus and Mary. Turn off the computer and the TV. Sit quietly in your room when you say your prayers. Carve out a special time in your day for you and Jesus. The Bible tells us in 1st Kings that the Lord comes to us not in loud noises such as thunder but in the "still small voice" and the soft winds. Instead of spending a lot of time looking into the mirror and judging yourself harshly, take time to look deep into your heart and to see yourself again as God sees you, a perfectly beautiful creation, and His creation.

"For you created my inmost being; you knit me together in my mother's womb. I praise you because I am fearfully and wonderfully made. Your works are wonderful. I know that full well."
Psalm 139:13-14

Stages and Changes

Between the ages of eight and fifteen you will begin to go through a stage called puberty, which will transform you from a little girl into a woman. This usually takes a couple of years. A large system in the body called the Endocrine System is producing chemicals called hormones that cause this change. There are many variations of how puberty may actually occur in one girl versus another but changes will take place in every single girl, in you and in your best friend. But no matter who you are, you will notice these things, as you become an adult.

Your breasts will begin to develop. Some girls notice a hard lump the size of a pea underneath the nipple. These are called breast buds. They may be tender to the touch. One girl described it as a "stick poking from the inside out." As time goes on, the area around the buds gets larger. Your breasts are a gift from God so that if you become a mother one day, your own body will be able to nourish your baby. It is important to practice modesty as your breasts develop by wearing a bra. Ask your mother to get you one or go shopping together.

Check out more information on bras in All Things Girl: Modern and Modest.

Stages and Changes

You will discover hair growth in your private area. This is called pubic hair. You will also begin to see hair under your arms and thicker hair on your legs. Pubic hair protects your intimate female parts. In this culture it is customary to remove hair from the underarms, and legs while in other cultures girls and women leave their hair alone. Remember that no matter what culture you live in and what customs you practice, God made everyone!

There are many hair removal methods to discuss with your mom. Some girls will shave their legs and underarms while others may wax or use a hair removal cream. The important thing is to never shave any part of your body or use a hair removal method unless you have discussed it with your mom. She will help you to know when hair removal is appropriate for you. Sometimes moms of lighter haired girls will want their daughters to wait while moms of darker haired girls may let their daughters remove hair at an earlier age. This is one of those times where mom knows best and God expects you to honor her! Plus, when you speak with your mom about these things, she will also see that you are growing up and will want to honor your interest in doing what is right.

Modesty protects the intimate center of the person. It means refusing to unveil what should remain hidden. CCC #2521

Stages and Changes

Part of the Endocrine System also includes sweat glands. Sweat glands increase production of sweat as a way to cool your body off. At the end of the day, you may notice that you smell like your dad after he mows the lawn (well maybe not that bad). You may also find that once you are in puberty you may sweat because you are nervous or anxious. All these things are natural and just mean that it is time to use deodorant. Deodorant keeps you fresh and clean smelling. You will want to put on deodorant right after your morning shower so you can keep that clean feeling all day long. Once you start sweating it may be too late for the deodorant so putting it on first thing in the morning is a good habit to add to your morning ritual (that should also include prayer – remember that from "Friends, Boys, and Getting Along?") Anyhow, deodorant comes in many forms: roll on, stick, gel, or spray. Choose one with mom that works best for you. It's a good idea to keep extra deodorant in your locker in case you need it.

Puberty also causes the oil glands to increase production. See Basic Skincare section for more information on caring for your skin.

Stages and Changes

Menstruation is a process that occurs every month and most women refer to it as their "period." The lining in the womb builds up a thick layer of blood and fluid. It is like a thick blanket to keep a baby warm. When the girl or woman is not married and there is no baby in the womb, this blanket is not needed so it will slough off and exit through the vagina. Somewhere between the ages of 8-16, girls experience their first period. It is a very important event in the life of a girl because it marks the transition from girlhood to womanhood.

Sometimes girls feel anxious about getting their period for the first time. There is no need to be nervous if you know what to expect. Some girls will notice a thick whitish discharge days or weeks before menstruation. Later this may be mixed with blood. You feel a wet sensation during your period. Mom and you can put together a girl's kit that you can keep in your purse, backpack or locker. Find a cute makeup bag and put some wipes, a pad, a change of undies, and a plastic ziplock baggie for soiled panties. This will give you confidence in case you get your first period when you are away from home. Some moms talk to the teacher and set up a code so that the girl can call home if she needs to talk to mom about her period if she is at school. For example, "I have a special visitor and need to call my mom," or "I don't feel well, I need to call my mom." If you don't feel comfortable doing that, remember that your girl's kit is a great way to be prepared for this special time in your life.

At first your period may not be regular, meaning it will not come at the same time every month. As time goes on though, it will happen once a month around the same day. You will need to get a calendar and mark this event so that you will know when to expect your period each month and be prepared with your supplies.

Talk to your mom and she will get you the feminine protection you need to feel fresh. Mom is the best person to help you when you get your period. She was once a girl your age and she knows how you feel. Talk to her about any concerns you have and she will make you feel better. Take a bath or shower daily during your period to stay fresh and clean. Try the bath salts recipe included in this book for something different.

Stages and Changes

PMS stands for premenstrual syndrome. It includes symptoms many girls experience before they get their period. You may have several or none at all. They include: bloating, cramps, breast tenderness, moodiness, breakout of pimples, headaches, tiredness, backaches and food cravings. Have your mom ask a doctor or pharmacist about taking a multivitamin and vitamin B complex. These can help ease PMS. Use a heating pad or take a hot bath or shower for cramps and backaches. Eat a lot of fruits, veggies, and protein and skip the junk food. Exercise helps too. If you find cramps keep you from normal activities, talk to your mom and have her take you to the doctor.

It is not unusual for a girl to feel like crying for no reason, having the urge to blow up, or to get her feelings hurt easily a week or so before her period. This is part of PMS. If you are keeping track on your calendar, you will notice when you can expect your period and be aware that this is why you are feeling sensitive. No matter what, it is important to remember you are in charge of how you react to things. Yes, PMS plays a part in your moods, but ultimately, you are responsible for your actions and reactions. Are you a drama queen?

For more information on emotions, get All Things Girl book, "Friends, Boys and Getting Along" where there is a section just on emotions.

Make These Yourself

Bath Salts

Try the salt when you need a little TLC and relax in your own private spa! These make great gifts too.

Ingredients and Directions:
Epsom salt
Essential oils, such as lavender, or orange
Food Coloring

Mix 1 cup of Epsom salt, ¼ cup sea salt, add 2-3 drops of essential oils, and food coloring to your preference. Add to bath water and enjoy!

Put the colored salt in jars. Decorate the jars with lace, sequences, or beads and give as a gift.

Skincare

Pore Strips

This mixture will clean your pores which when clogged cause blackheads or pimples.

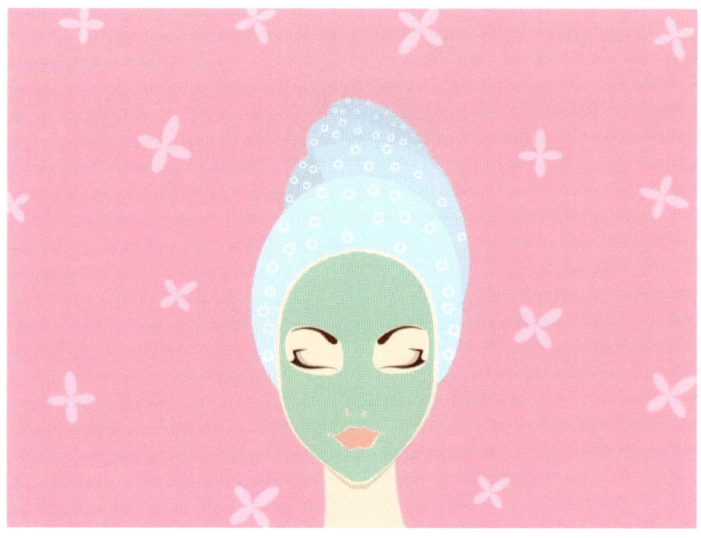

Ingredients and Directions:

1 Tablespoon of plain unsweetened gelatin (look in the isle where Jello is sold) and 1½ Tablespoon of milk

Mix the two ingredients in a bowl. Heat until it forms a paste. Apply the mixture to parts of the face such as nose, chin, or forehead where blackheads and pimples appear. Let dry. Remove and look. You will see how much "yuck" was in your pores!

Sunburn Relief Ingredients and Directions:

1 small grated potato (peeled); 2-3 Teaspoons of flour; Water

Mix the ingredients, adding enough flour and water to make it the consistency of cake batter. Spread over the burned area. Leave on the face for 20-30 minutes. Rinse with water.

Lip Exfoliant for Dry, Flaky Lips Ingredients and Directions:

Ingredients; Sugar; Olive Oil

Mix equal parts of the above ingredients. Apply to the lips rubbing gently back and forth. This will remove dry skin leaving your lips soft and moisturized. Rinse with water.

As a hair stylist, and fashion consultant, I learned techniques to help others look and feel their best. I am passing on to you the tricks of the trade so that you, as a daughter of the King, will always look your best!

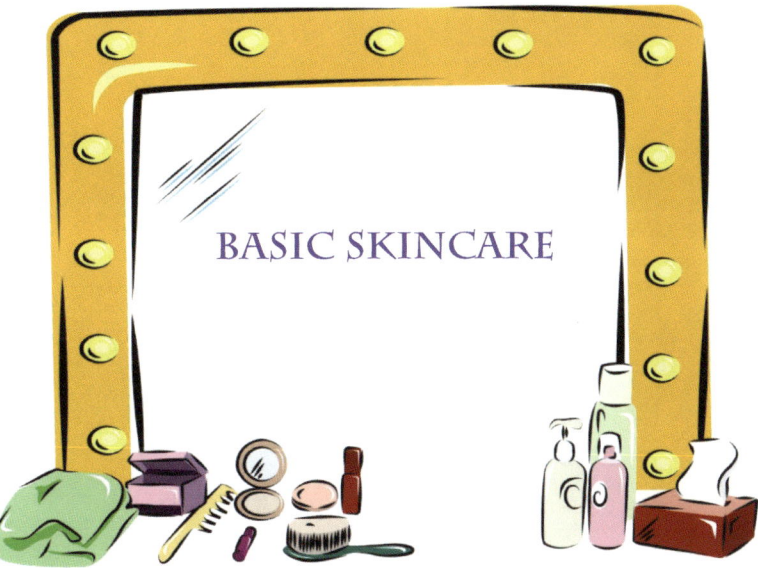

BASIC SKINCARE

The skin is the largest organ of the body. It is the only organ that can be "regulated." This means, that by changing products or habits, it will act differently. The skin keeps the organs and muscles protected from the outside world. Breakouts and rashes are impurities being purged from the inside.

During puberty, hormones are changing and producing more oil. This can cause blemishes or blackheads. Besides caring for the skin, there are a few other things that can be done to keep breakouts under control:

- Shower and shampoo frequently
- Change pillowcase daily (if this makes a lot of wash for mom, offer to help with laundry)
- Use clean towels and washcloths (if this makes a lot of wash for mom, offer to help with laundry)
- Limit or avoid greasy foods
- Limit or avoid sugar and white flour intake
- Limit or avoid dairy intake
- Increase vegetable and fruit intake
- Drink lots of water to help the skin eliminate impurities

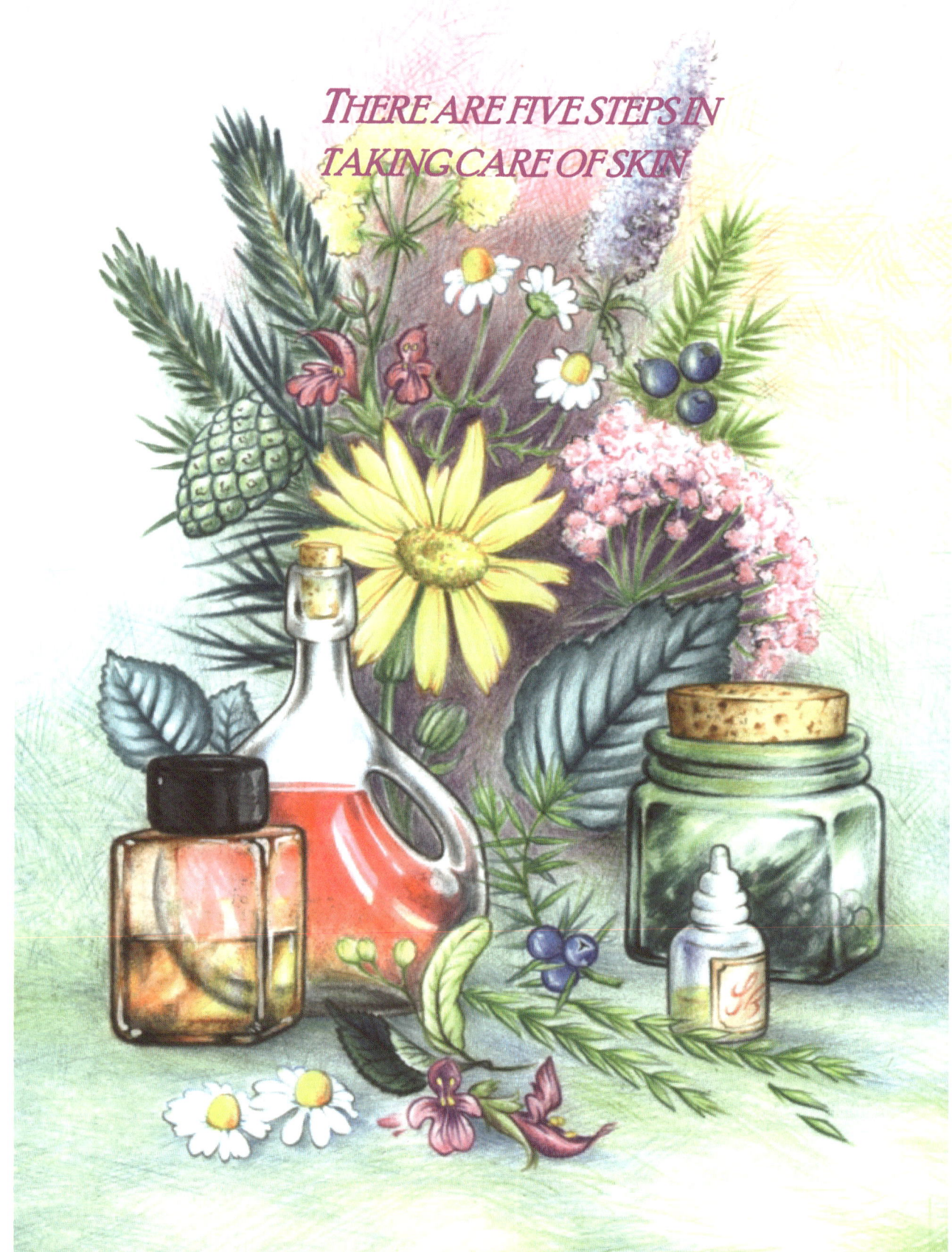

Step 1: Cleanse the Face

Use a gentle and water soluble cleanser. The worst thing to use is soap and water. This will dry out the skin and send a signal to the oil glands to produce more oil. Many teenagers feel their skin is not clean unless it feels tight or tingly. This is a myth. Most soaps not only dry the skin but have ingredients that clog pores. Use upward and outward motions to clean your face. You can use a soft washcloth with cleanser on it, or your fingers. Rinse with cool water after cleansing.

Step 2: Exfoliating

This step will remove dead skin particles that can clog pores. In doing this the newer, healthier skin surfaces. A topical, mechanical scrub is best if it is extremely fine. Over-scrubbing can break open blemishes or cause abrasions. It is important to be gentle when using a scrub. Again, use upward and outward motions with either your fingers or cloth. Avoid the eye area. Rinse clean with cool water. Those with acne should not use a scrub. The other option for exfoliating is Alpha Hydroxy or Beta Hydroxy, which are mild chemicals that slough the skin without using a scrub. They are available in many skincare product lines.

Step 3: Tone

Use a toner to make the skin feel clean and smooth. Benzoyl peroxide is considered the best over the counter drug to use in fighting blemishes. If you do not have blemishes do not use a toner. It is not necessary if you have done a good job cleansing. Toners can dry the skin if they are not needed.

Step 4 & 5: Moisturize and Protect

Everyone needs to moisturize the skin, even if you have oily skin. A light moisturizer will help regulate the oil production. Protect the skin by using a SPF 15 or greater. By staying out of the sun, the skin will be less damaged and look younger longer. When you are old enough to wear makeup, a foundation is part of the protection step. There are a variety of foundation types to choose from such as cream foundation, cream to powder, mineral powder and liquid.

OTHER SKIN CONSIDERATIONS

It's a good idea to use high quality products for skincare and makeup. Many companies produce good items. Girls your age often like to take advice from each other about skincare and makeup, however, their advice is most likely unreliable at best. To find the right products at good prices, mom needs to do some research. Some companies have home classes so that you can try before you buy. This is highly recommended.

If breakouts become frequent and cover a large area of the face, it's a good idea to have mom take you to the doctor. Unless you get a referral from your pediatrician or family doctor, there is no need to start with a dermatologist. Many times a low dose of an antibiotic or medicated topical cream will clear up the breakout.

Going to an esthetician can also help with blemishes. They are trained in skincare and techniques to deep clean the skin.

When you are old enough to wear makeup, which is up to your mother, it is important to learn proper techniques to use makeup to enhance your face, not to cover it up. Many young girls resemble Cleopatra, which detracts from their natural beauty. Being a daughter of the King, you want to look your best. However, physical beauty is only skin deep while your inner beauty is what makes you the person you are and is the most important thing.

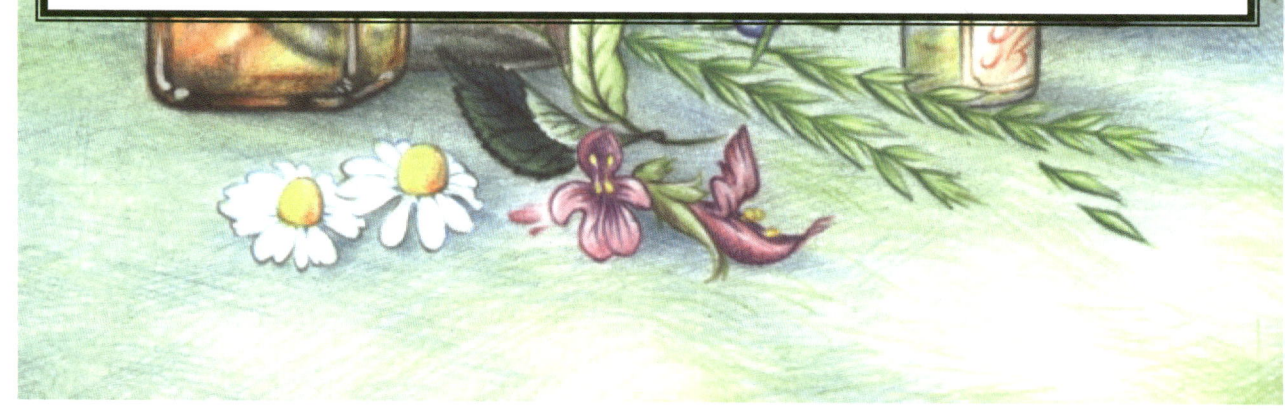

Hair

There are many things for a girl to pay attention to when it comes to looking good. Beauty is something that our culture emphasizes. Though a girl must take care to always look her best, it is important not to get carried away. It is not good to spend large amounts of time in front of the mirror. Young women have to work at finding a balance so as not to become self-centered. Remember, everyone has God given beauty and realizing this is important because it helps you to overcome the culture's view of beauty and recognize God's view of beauty and dignity. Embrace your uniqueness. You are a princess, a daughter of the King and are worth more than a rare jewel!

This is the time to learn to love and accept how God has made you so your whole life can be filled with the joy that comes from that knowledge.

Your hair is one of the things to consider when you want to look your best. Before you even try to decide what hairstyle is best for you, though, make sure you are taking good care of your hair. At your age, it is important to shampoo your hair every day to avoid that greasy look. The best kind of shampoo is a clarifying shampoo followed by a light conditioner. Clarifying means a shampoo that deep cleans and gets rid of build up of products like mousse or gel or hairspray. Even if you don't use products like that, a clarifying shampoo really deep cleans. Remember that puberty is a time where sweat and oil glands are working overtime and that means you will even notice it in your hair.

THERE ARE MANY BEAUTY SUPPLY STORES WHERE YOU CAN FIND LARGE SIZES OF SALON SHAMPOO AND CONDITIONER. IF YOU DON'T KNOW OF ONE IN YOUR AREA, YOU COULD PROBABLY FIND ONE IN THE PHONE BOOK.

It is recommended that you use a salon shampoo and conditioner. It costs a little more, but you don't have to use much and it lasts a long time. As you grow into a woman you will realize that there is a price tag on quality products. However, in a family there is only so much money to spend on all the needs of the family. Shampoo and conditioner from the salon may seem like a luxury. Deciding priorities is an important part of growing up and talking with your mom about these things is a part of the growing up process. Together you and your mom can determine priorities for your beauty regimen and you can help make those priorities happen by saving your babysitting money or doing without an extra pair of jeans. Let your mom see that you care not only about yourself but about the family.

Anyhow, five liters of salon shampoo lasts about a year for a family of five. Use about a dime size or so every time you shampoo your hair. Use conditioner the same way. Professional shampoo may not lather up but not to worry, it's working. Professional products don't build up on the hair like drugstore shampoos do. This is what causes hair to look greasy by noon, even if you showered and shampooed your hair that very morning.

With your mom, check it out: take a sharp scissors and scrape the blade over a small chunk of hair in an upward motion. If you have been using inexpensive shampoo and conditioner, you will see a white buildup on the blade. This is balsam. It' like candle wax and is an ingredient in nonprofessional products. Once you begin using quality hair products you will notice a difference in how your hair feels and how it styles.

More on Hair...
Keep on getting trims about every six weeks to keep those locks lovely!

Do you like to swim? Make sure you shampoo after each swim. Chlorine can build up in the hair and ruin your beautiful locks. If your hair is full of chlorine it will appear very shiny and sometimes have a touch of green to the color. When wet, it will feel like cooked spaghetti. You can do a clarifying treatment at the salon or at home to help strip the chlorine. Purchase the clarifying product, shampoo hair, apply product, cover with a plastic bag and let it sit for 15-30 minutes. Rinse and apply a light conditioner. Don't forget the conditioner or your hair will be a total rat's nest! The clarifier opens the hair shaft and pulls out the impurities, leaving the strand open, which causes tangles.

When combing out long hair, start at the part line and work in small sections, combing down. This will keep your hair from breaking. (Ever hear your hair snap, crackle and pop? It's hair breakage.) Combing this way will result in nice smooth hair.

If you are thinking about a perm, its best to wait until after you get your first period. Hormones can do funny things to hair and oftentimes perms do not "take" on children. That means they don't do what they are supposed to do.

Dandruff is something girls may or may not experience. Dandruff refers to a flaky scalp. It may be caused by several things. First, the scalp may be dry which will cause flakes and itching. Secondly, the scalp may be oily and the flakes may be large oily flakes. Next, shampoo and other products may not be rinsed out and this causes flakes of products, not the skin. Whatever the cause, the best way to be rid of dandruff is to use a coal tar shampoo every day until you get the problem under control. Then you may go back to using the clarifying shampoo. Coal tar shampoo can be found in a pharmacy. It doesn't smell very good, but, boy it works!

Girls often make the mistake of copying movie stars or fashion models when picking a hairstyle for themselves. Why is this a mistake? Well, you are unique. You have different hair and features than the famous people on TV, in magazines, or in the movies. Their stylists work hard to find the best hair design just for them. Problem is, girls mimic these styles, even if these styles look awful on them or just aren't right.

Here are some things to consider when deciding which style is just right for you:

~FACE SHAPE~

If you are unsure what your face shape is, pull back your hair and look in the mirror. You can also ask your hairstylist to help you decide which shape you are.

~FACIAL FEATURES~

With your hair pulled back decide what is your best feature for example your eyes or your smile. You will want to emphasize this. Always accentuate the positive. If you have a prominent nose, choose something that is not straight and flat.

~LIFE STYLE~

Think about how much you will really work with your hair. How active are you in sports? Do you like wearing hair accessories such as barrettes? It's not a good idea to have a style with lots of layers if you won't style it or you play on a sports team and need to keep your hair out of your face. It just won't work

~HAIR TYPE~

Is your hair thick or thin? Straight or curly? Do you have cowlicks that make your hair hard to style? If you have curly hair, you will not be able to wear a straight, flat-layered style. Learn early it's best to work with the hair you have, not fight against it.

~TIME~

How much time do you plan to spend on your hair? Are you willing to get up early before school to blow dry and style it?

~Cost~

How often will you need a trim to keep the style? How much money is your mom willing to spend to keep up your hairstyle? What are the family priorities? Again, the family has expenses for all the members. You may have to choose between keeping up your hair or a new pair of shoes. It's not all about you, but about learning how to pick and choose what it most important. You may have to make an arrangement with mom that you pay for some things with your hard earned babysitting money.

Consider all of these things when choosing a hairstyle. Remember, as a daughter of the King it is important to take care of your personal appearance, but how you treat people and what is inside is much more important.

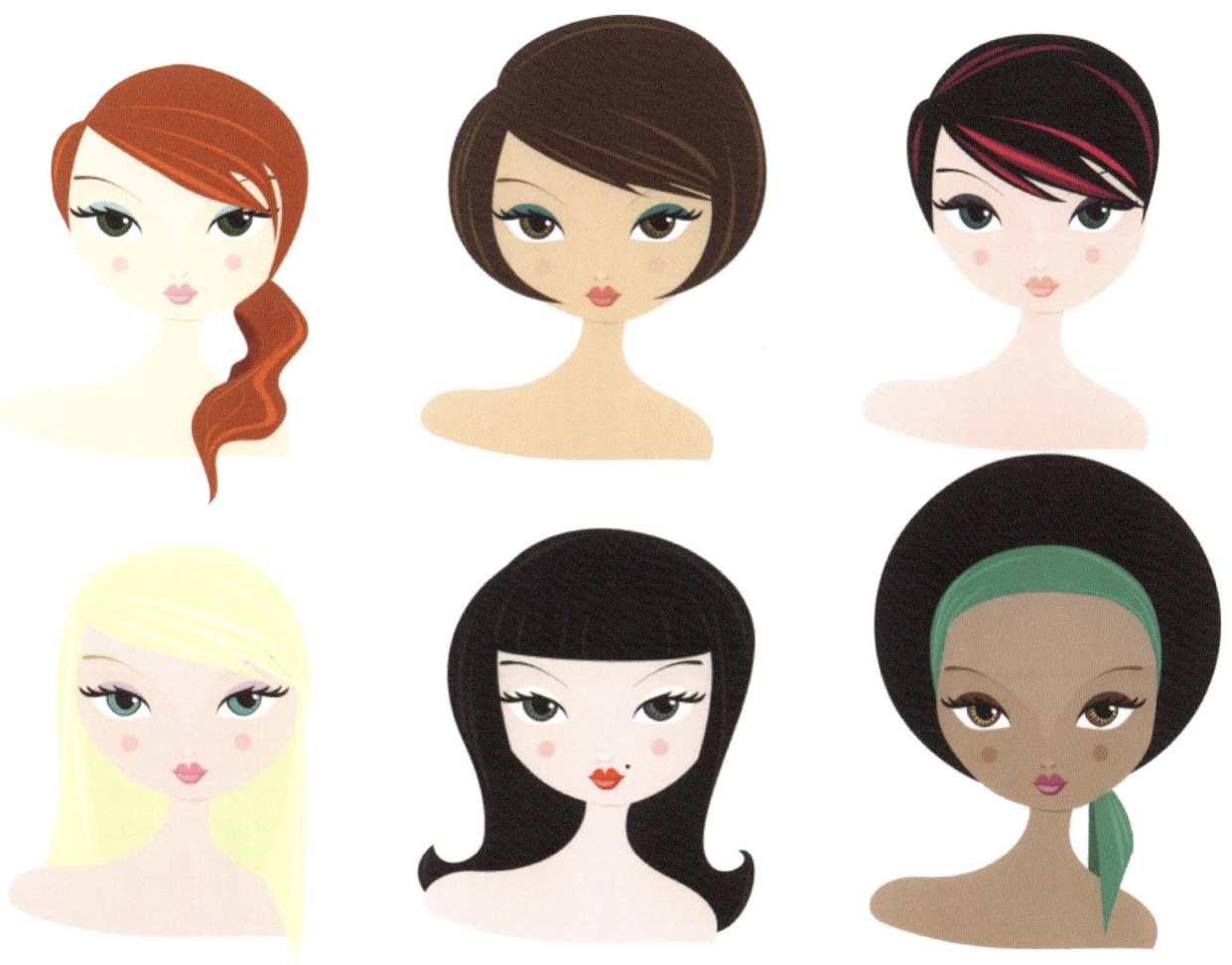

There are a number of styling aids on the market today. Just like shampoo and conditioner, it is best to use the professional brands from a salon. Many inexpensive brands flake, buildup, or dry out the hair. Remember, a little dab will do ya! The hair industry, like fashion, is constantly changing and you will see new products all the time. However, below is a list of basic styling products. Choose the ones that are right for you.

- **MOUSSE: USED TO GIVE BODY AND FULLNESS**
    - Squirt about the size of a quarter into your hand and rub your palms together.
    - After the foam is like a lotion, apply to the wet hair shaft.

- **GEL: GIVES HOLDING POWER**
    - Apply gel the size of a dime or nickel into your hand and rub the palms together.
    - Apply the gel to the wet hair shaft closest to the scalp and pull through.

- **THERMAL SPRAY: HELPS WHEN STYLING WITH HEAT, LIKE CURLING IRON OR BLOW DRYER**
    - Can be used on wet or dry hair.

- **POMADE: HELPS TO DEFINE A DRY STYLE BY SEPARATING PIECES OF HAIR.**
    - Apply a very small amount to the palms and pull through the hair shaft.
    - Use fingers to "piece out" your hairstyle.

- **SHINING SOLUTIONS: COME IN SPRAY OR GEL FORM MADE FROM SILICONE**
    -Apply to styled hair, very conservatively.

- **HAIR SPRAYS:**
    - Aerosol: Comes in a can and sprays a mist. It varies in holding power from a working hold to a "cement hold".
    - Non-aerosol: Comes in a bottle with a spray top. Varies in holding power but comes out in a wet mist.

- **CURLS:** There are many products for curly hair to help straighten or smooth. Always ask your hairdresser for the newest options. The hair care industry changes rapidly and is always bringing forth new products.

Face Shape	Try	Avoid
Oval Gently rounded hairline with a slightly narrower jaw than temples	-Short, medium or long hairstyles -Textured layers or bangs -This shape is balanced and can wear a variety of styles	-Heavy bangs and forward styled hair because it covers the face and can add weight.
Triangular Dominant jaw line and narrow cheekbones and temples	-Shorter, fuller hair at the top and narrowing at the jaw -Off center parts -Wedges and shags are good -Tuck hair behind the ears	-Long, full hairstyles that draw attention to the full jaw line -Center parts -Long straight hair, no bangs
Round Full face, round chin and hairline with widest point at the cheeks	-Styles with fullness and height at the crown and front -Off center parts -Short hairstyles styled off the face -Medium lengths past the chin -Layered top -Close to the face cuts	-Chin length cuts -Center parts -Very short hair -Fullness at the cheekbone
Square Strong jaw line, square hairline	-Short and medium cuts -Loose curls and waves around the face -Wispy bangs, razored sides to soften face -Height at the crown -Angle cut bobbed cuts with razored edges, above the jaw line	-Long straight styles -Straight, boxy bangs -Straight cut bob
Heart Wide temples and hairline with a small chin	-Weighted cut at the chin, like a bob -Side swept bangs -Soft razored bangs or none at all -Flipped up shag with longer layers on the top	-Short full styles, height at the crown -Top heavy styles

Makeup Application

When you are old enough to wear makeup, and this is up to mom, it's important to know what you're doing. Always remember makeup enhances your already beautiful face and young skin. Some girls your age are allowed to wear lipgloss and sparkly powder. Later in your teens, when mom gives the okay you will want to experiment with other makeup. Here are some tried and true basics that makeup artists from all over the world use.   Always apply make up to a clean face!

Step 1: Concealer

Use to cover blemishes, dark circles or other flaws; Choose a shade at least two shades lighter than your skin; Use a sponge applicator and dab on skin; Do not pull or tug the skin

Step 2: Foundation

Choose a foundation EXACTLY your skin color; Use a foundation with at least SPF 15; Choose foundation to go with your skin type (ex: oil free, cream to powder or liquid); Use a sponge applicator and dab makeup in spots all over face and eye lids
Blend in gently in an outward motion; Don't apply under the chin or on the neck

Step 3: Powder

Use a large natural hair brush to apply loose or pressed powder; Tap brush on the edge of the container to knock off the excess; Apply in a downward motion

Step 4: Eye Makeup

There are many techniques to use with different eye shapes. The following application works for all shapes; Use natural hair eye shadow brush; Knock excess powder; Apply lightest shadow from brow to lashes; Select a darker shade in the same color family and apply to the crease and eyelid; Use a darker brown, charcoal or black to line the upper lash line only. If you line lower, it will close in the eye; Apply mascara from bottom of lashes to the top. Do not "pump" the tube. Discard mascara tube after 6-12 weeks to avoid eye infections

Step 5: Eyebrow arch

Follow the natural arch of the brow; Fill in the brow with a natural brown eye shadow that matches. Shadow is softer than a pencil; The end of the brow should end at the corner of the eye; As a side note, tweeze or wax stray brows for a clean, finished look. Do not make them too thin. Stay with the natural arch.

Step 6: Blush

Blush is applied to give contour to the face, not for "rosy cheeks"; Use a natural hair brush if using a powder and knock off excess; If using a cream or liquid, use your fingers or a sponge, apply a couple dots and blend from end of nose at the outside corner of the eye, underneath the cheek bone, near the hair line, toward the ear; Apply powder the same way

Step 7: Lipstick and Lip liner

Always use a lip liner; Use short, feathery strokes to outline the lips
Choose a liner in the same color family as the lipstick; Fill in with lip liner and go over with lipstick; Using lip brush will make your application cleaner; Add gloss

Nails

You wouldn't be completely groomed without having your nails manicured. Many people talk with their hands so it is important to take care of them. What's more unattractive than a girl with dirty nails? Well, maybe a girl with nails bitten down to the nub!

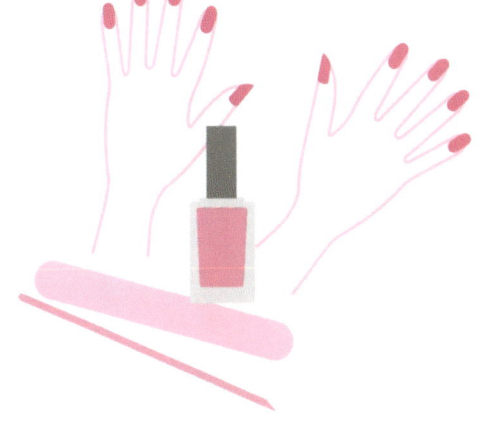

You don't have to spend lots of money at a nail salon to have nice hands. There are a few steps the professionals use and you can, too. Check it out below.

If you are a nail biter, chances are it is a nervous habit and can be broken. There are remedies that taste awful you can get at the drugstore to help break the habit. Do it now when you are young so that it doesn't follow you into adulthood. Take a little time to notice when you start biting and see if you can consciously make a change. If something is bothering you talk to your mother or another trusted adult.

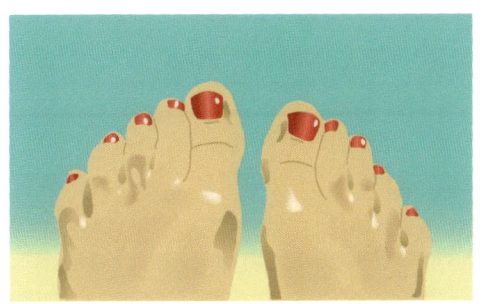

Summer is a time for pretty sandals and flip-flops. Better get those tootsies looking good by getting a pedicure. Just like having steps for a manicure there are basic steps professionals use for a pedicure that you can learn too. This is a fun thing to do with mom, sisters and friends.

Manicure and Pedicure

MATERIALS NEEDED:

- Containers to soak feet
- Bowls to soak hands
- Towels to dry feet and hands
- Cuticle remover
- Nail polish remover
- A cuticle pusher, which is also called an orangewood stick
- Nippers cut off hang nails (because you should never bite them!)
- Emery boards
- Mild, disinfectant soap
- Pedi-file
- Exfoliator or scrub to remove dead skin
- Polish
- Decals
- Mini-polishes with tiny brushes to make designs (Sally's Beauty Supply)

MANICURE STEPS AT HOME

Step 1; Soak hands in warm, mild soapy water.

Step 2; Apply cuticle remover, push back and trim cuticles with nippers.

Step 3; Shape the nail with a nail file. To remove length, use a coarser file.

Step 4; Apply base coat.

Step 5; Apply polish. Always polish in three strokes, starting in the center and then each side.

Step 6; Apply topcoat.

Step 7; Clean up around the cuticle if needed.

Nail shapes

SQUARE   OVAL   POINTED

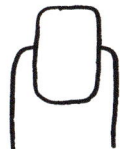 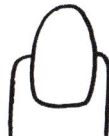 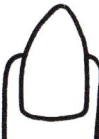

PEDICURE STEPS AT HOME

Step 1; Soak feet in warm, soapy water.

Step 2; Apply exfoliating lotion and massage in. (Various products such as salts and sugars can also be used)

Step 3; Use pedi-file to remove dead skin.

Step 4; Rinse feet.

Step 5; Apply cuticle remover; push back and trim cuticles.

Step 6; Clip toenails giving the nails a square shape. File if necessary to smooth.

Step 7; Apply emollient lotion

Step 8; Apply nail polish remover to the toenails to remove lotion.

Steps 9, 10, 11; Apply base coat, polish and topcoat. Apply in three strokes starting in the middle.

Step 12; Remove excess polish with remover.

A daughter of the King looks her best at all times to give glory to her Father.

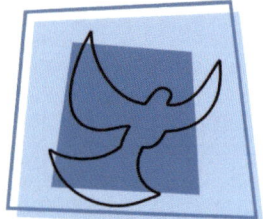

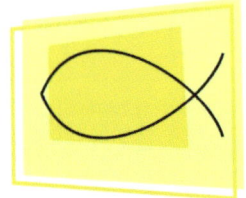

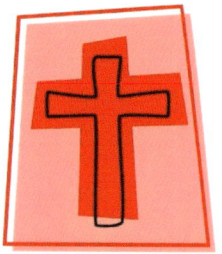

With all these beauty tips, you may be thinking these things take hours. Daily routines of basic hygiene such as showering, brushing and flossing teeth, and skincare take only a few minutes once you get in the habit. Hairstyling and applying makeup, take more time. This is the time when you have to be considerate of others in the family so that you do not take over the bathroom. It takes a little time to get your habits down to a science. The idea is to get your daily grooming done in a reasonable amount of time so that you do not become self-centered. Many women can get ready for the day in 30 minutes, including a shower.

Being part of the culture today does not mean being self-absorbed but looking beautiful as is customary in today's society. Taking care of your appearance is an outward sign of knowing your worth as a person and embracing the fact that you are a princess.

True Beauty, Inner Beauty

Do you remember reading fairy tale books or watching movies of Cinderella, Snow White, and Belle? All of them have beautiful faces and hair, not to mention a perfect figure. Take a minute and think of what else they have in common. They are kind, cheerful, generous, compassionate and forgiving. That's what makes them truly beautiful.

Lots of girls your age think that being pretty is the most important thing. However, that is not what is going to bring you love and true happiness. Think of all the popular singers and stars of today. They have talent and outward attractiveness but, sadly, many of them have miserable lives. In the end what did all that beauty do for them? Let's not diminish the fact that most girls want to be cute. But it does take a little growing up to see that there's more to attractiveness than meets the eye. Have you ever had a friend that you just loved but she was plain looking, chubby, or had bad skin? Something made you want to be with her and get to know her. That is called inner beauty. That which you cannot see is attractive to you and you want to have a friendship with that person. Confidence is part of inner beauty. Did you ever wonder what was the source of inner confidence?

Well, it comes from your Heavenly Father. God has stamped dignity on your heart and to Him you are His precious daughter and your beauty is beyond compare. The Bible says that man looks at the outside but God looks at the heart. A person can be considered "good looking," but have an "ugly" soul because of a sinful heart or mean spirit. To have true beauty, inner beauty, it's important to be kind to others, be cheerful, share your things, forgive easily, and to imitate Jesus and His Blessed Mother as much as you can. Look around you. Most of the time people with lots of friends are easy to get along with and do the things just mentioned. While it is important as the daughter of the King to look your best, it's much more important to act your best. Spend more energy on your inner beauty. You'll be glad you did!

Virtues to Live by...

What is a virtue? Very simply, a virtue is a good habit that inclines you to do whatever is good. Virtuous behavior helps you live a good, happy life. But there is more to virtues than that. A single good action does not constitute a virtue. For instance, a person wouldn't be considered to have the virtue of generosity if she shared her candy with her friends only once. In order to become a virtue, a good habit has to be repeated on a regular basis.

Humility

Humility is recognizing and acknowledging your true position with respect to God and other people. It means looking at yourself as you really are, honestly and without excuses. It means accepting that you depend absolutely on God: without Him, you can do nothing, you are nothing.

If you are humble, you avoid bragging about your accomplishments; instead, you turn to God in thanksgiving for all the wonderful things He has accomplished through you. A humble person recognizes the talents of others and is not envious about it. She knows when to ask for advice, recognizing that she doesn't know everything. This is super important when your parents try to help you and give you advice: remember, they once were your age and have way more experience in life than you, so if you are humble, you will not take the attitude of: "I know it all."

The opposite of humility is pride, which is an excessive love and admiration of self. A proud person thinks she is superior to others. She sees her talents or looks as something she acquired on her own, instead of as gifts from God.. A proud person tries to attract notice, praise, and seeks to be the center of attention. A proud person compares herself to others and considers herself better thinking to herself: "I'm much better at volleyball than she is...."

Some girls are proud of their appearance. This is called vanity. Mirror, mirror on the wall, who is the fairest one of all? Remember the queen in Snow White, asking –forcing– the mirror to acknowledge her as the most beautiful? She is a perfect example of vanity! The best way to combat vanity is to recall that God has made you just as you are and has given you all that you need. God gave you a certain eye, hair color, family, talents, etc. Each is a gift from God that He can take away at any time.

Here are some possible goals to help you be humble:

- When you find yourself thinking about your great accomplishments, give them to God and thank Him for giving you talents.
- Avoid spending too much time looking at yourself in the mirror aka, primping.
- When somebody gives you words of praise, thank them and tell yourself, it's all from God.
- Avoid comparing yourself to others.
- Be graceful when you fail: accept your defeats and mistakes.
- Give God the credit for all the good in your life.
- Accept positive criticism from your parents and friends cheerfully.
- Admit when you did something wrong and learn to apologize.

Things to Think About

an examination of conscience for girls

- Do I always have to be the center of attention?
- Do I think of my talents and beauty as things that I achieved for myself?
- How much time do I spend in front of the mirror?
- Am I a good sport when I lose?
- Do I take constructive criticism with a good attitude?
- Do I want to be first in everything?
- Do I apologize when I have done wrong?
- Do I admit my mistakes?
- Do I insist on wearing only the best and most stylish clothing?
- Do I judge others by how they look and by what they wear?
- Am I a bragger?
- Am I jealous of others' looks or accomplishments?

Am I Vain?

Now that you know about the virtue humility and the vice (bad habit) of vanity, take the quiz to see which you are.

At a party I like to:

a) be the center of attention
b) sit back and watch everything
c) listen and butt in when I have something to add to the conversation or activity

When I get a new outfit, I:

a) go to school and expect everyone to notice and give me a compliment
b) quietly wear my outfit and don't expect to be noticed
c) proudly wear my outfit and thank those who give me a compliment

When I get ready for school or to go someplace, I:

a) make sure I am the first in the bathroom and take at least an hour to make sure I look great
b) get dressed and do my normal grooming quickly so that my family doesn't have to wait on me
c) get dressed and ready taking my time until someone tells me they need the bathroom

When my friends come over we like to:

a) get out all the makeup, nail polish and hair products we can and lock ourselves in the bathroom trying everything on each other
b) listen to music, make cookies, or do crafts
c) do crafts, play ball, bike ride, do manicure and pedicures

Whenever I pass a mirror, I:

a) sneak a peak to make sure my face, hair, and clothes are perfect
b) don't really notice mirrors
c) check my appearance if I notice

Whenever I get a compliment, I:

a) am proud of myself and feel I deserve it
b) accept it with a grateful heart knowing my gifts are from God
c) thank the person giving me the compliment and feel proud

Whenever my parents give me correction, I:

a) argue and roll my eyes figuring they don't know anything.
b) listen and think about what they are saying and apologize
c) listen with anger and stomp off, later apologizing for my wrong doing

When I am asked to apologize, I:

a) roll my eyes and refuse
b) feel bad about my mistake and beg to be forgiven
c) reluctantly admit my mistake and apologize

Key

Mostly a's: Girl, you need a dose of humility! The world does not revolve around you. Take time to think about the virtue of humility and think of a small way to begin being humble. For example, try taking less time getting ready for the day. Your beauty and gifts come from your Heavenly Father. Thank Him and *Rock On!*

Mostly b's: What a wonder you are! You have discovered the beauty of humility. Thank your Father in Heaven and keep on keeping on!

Mostly c's: You're getting there sister, but like the rest of us, you can learn to be a bit more humble. Every day try to do something concrete to get better at humility such as not interrupting a conversation others are having.

YOU'VE GOTTA HAVE A PLAN!

You know it is important to take care of and control your body. In the same way, you need to take care of your soul. You need to nourish it so that it can grow in friendship with Jesus. How is that done? You gotta have a plan!

Do you think athletes make it to the Olympics by chance? Do you think they go with the flow and train here and there and somehow one day they end up in the Olympic games winning a medal? Of course not, you know that! They have a plan that includes diet and training. They follow it everyday, even when they don't feel like it. This dedication allows the athlete to attain their goal, their dream of winning a medal at the Olympics.

Think about the purpose of your life, to know, love and serve God in this life and to be happy with Him forever in the next. Do you think you can achieve this goal without some planning and preparation?

Here's a simple but effective plan you can use your entire life to complete your training here and attain your Heavenly goal. You can also use the special "All Things Girl" journal to write your own plan, prayers, and thoughts.

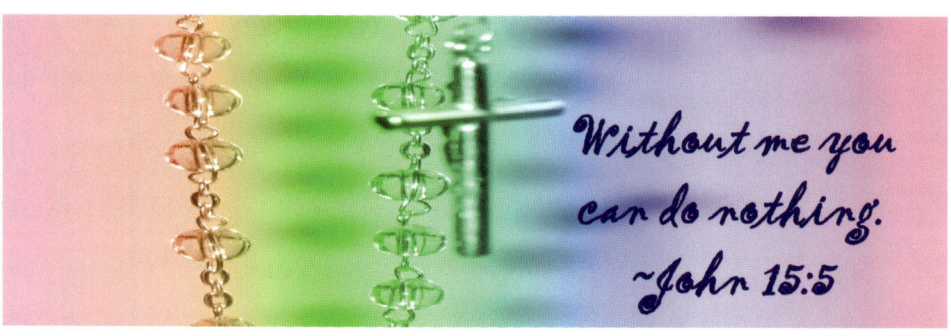

Without me you can do nothing.
~John 15:5

It's All Part of the Plan

WHAT THINGS SHOULD BE PART OF YOUR PLAN?

MORNING OFFERING:

A good way to start your day is to say, "Hello, Jesus!" The day ahead is a great gift from God. The morning offering consists of giving Jesus everything you will do and say that day. Tell Him you want to please Him and give Him glory in all that you do.

You can make up your own special prayer or you can choose one to memorize. For example, here's a very simple prayer.

"Good Morning dear Jesus this day is for you, I ask you to bless all that I say and do. Amen"

Or

"Oh Jesus through the Immaculate Heart of Mary I offer you the prayers, works, joys, and sufferings of this day, For all the intentions of Your Sacred Heart, in union with the Holy Sacrifice of the Mass said throughout the world today, in reparation for my sins, for the intentions of all our associates, and for the intentions of the Holy Father this month. Amen"

It is important to try and say your morning offering at the same time every day so that you remember to do it. Some girls will say it right when they wake up. Others, when they sit down to breakfast. Whatever works for you, just do it!

DAILY PRAYER.
Prayer is talking to Jesus. It is something great! Jesus prayed and openly encouraged his disciples to pray. And guess what? You, as a daughter of the King, are a disciple. How does a person learn to pray? Start out by setting aside 5 minutes of your day to sit down in a quiet place where there will be no distractions. Place yourself in the presence of Jesus, asking your guardian angel to help you start a conversation with Jesus. Because prayer is an intimate conversation with God, you can talk to God as your best friend and tell Him the things that are concerning you, what is making you happy, angry or sad; God is always listening. You may tell Him something like: *"Hi Jesus, guess what I'm doing today? I'm going to my cousins' house! Mom said I have to clean my room before going....and you know Jesus, I hate cleaning my room! But I guess I'll do it.... Maybe I should offer it up for a special intention, eh? Who needs prayers, Jesus?....."* On you go. You are praying! Slowly

increase the 5 minutes of prayer a day to 10 minutes. You will feel so happy when you spend time talking to Jesus every day!

THE ROSARY OF THE BLESSED MOTHER. Do you enjoy looking at family pictures and remembering those precious moments? Well, when you pray the rosary you contemplate moments in the lives of Jesus and Mary on each mystery. The rosary is divided into 4 parts: each part into five mysteries. For each mystery one Our Father and Ten Hail Mary's are prayed while you meditate on a certain time of Jesus' life. The name rosary means "crown of roses". Think about each of the Hail Mary's you pray as a rose offered to Our Lady. By the end of the rosary, you have offered her a huge bouquet of beautiful roses! If saying the entire rosary seems like a big task, start out with just one decade and slowly add one at a time. The idea is to make the effort and to keep on trying.

EXAMINATION OF CONSCIENCE AT NIGHT. Before going to bed, it's a good idea to take a quick look at your day in God's presence to see if you have behaved as a daughter of the King. An easy way to do this is by asking yourself these three questions:

- *What did I do today that was pleasing to God?*
- *What did I do today that was not pleasing to God?*
- *What does God want me to do better tomorrow?*

Ponder briefly on each question, and then follow with an act of contrition to tell Jesus that you are sorry for having offended Him. An Act of Contrition is just a short prayer telling Jesus you are sorry for your sins. It can be as simple as *"I'm sorry, Lord. Help me do better tomorrow."* Or it can be the traditional Act of Contrition, " *Oh my God, I am heartily sorry for having offended thee and I detest all my sins because of the loss of Heaven and the pains of Hell, But most of all because they offend Thee my God who are all good and deserving of all my love. I firmly resolve with the help of Thy grace, to confess my sins, to do penance and to amend my life, Amen."*

PRAY THREE HAIL MARY'S AT NIGHT BEFORE GOING TO BED ASKING THE BLESSED MOTHER TO HELP YOU KEEP YOUR HEART PURE.

Don't delay, start today, you can win the Olympics of the spiritual life!

A GIRL LIKE ME!

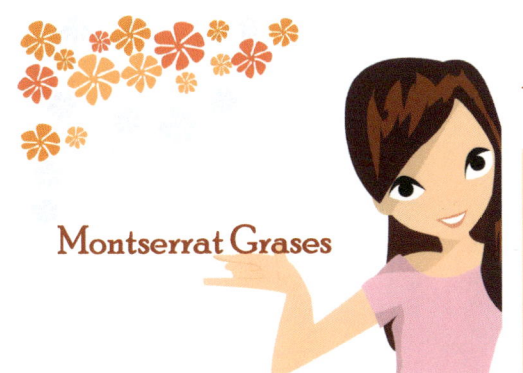

Montserrat Grases

Montserrat Grases was born in Barcelona, Spain, in 1941. Montse, as she was known by everyone, was the second of nine children.. Hers was a happy Christian family, where the older children helped take care of the home and younger children.

From the time she was little, Montse had a lively character: she was cheerful, very playful, always thinking up new games to play with her siblings. Her parents taught her and her siblings simple prayers to Jesus, the Blessed Mother and the Guardian Angel. They also taught her to accept and offer pain and sickness, and to tell the truth always.

Montse had a very happy childhood. She loved to play cops and robbers with her siblings and neighborhood friends; She was not born holy, but she became very holy as she grew up.

As a young teenager, Montse was a beautiful girl; she had a beautiful smile and she was very athletic. She had lots of friends and loved to go out with them. In school, she was one of the best students in the class, but she had great humility in never bragging about how smart she was. Also, she was very good at basketball, tennis and ping-pong.

At the age of 16, Montse felt that God was calling her to follow a way of sanctification (reaching holiness) in ordinary life in Opus Dei. She decided to give her life to God by living a plan for her spiritual life, similar to the one in this book, by offering to God all her activities, work and study and by bringing other people closer to Jesus. She spent time every day in prayer, conversing with Jesus about all sorts of things; she prayed the Holy Rosary, did an examination of conscience every night and had great devotion to Jesus in the Eucharist. All these things, prepared her soul for what God was going to ask from her at such a young age.

In January of 1958, when Montse was 16 years old, she went skiing with a group of friends. She fell and injured her leg. At the time, she didn't give it too much importance. She continued her life as normal but in a lot of pain. Montse thought her pain was a result from the fall. After several weeks, she decided to see the doctor, who told her to wear a kneepad, and let her leg rest as much as possible. This made Montse feel very sad. She enjoyed helping her mom around the house and taking care of her siblings. But she chose to be cheerful and offered her pain and frustration up to Jesus.

A couple of months later the pain in Montse's leg continued to increase. The doctor recommended putting a cast on her leg, which they did. This caused worse pain and discomfort for Montse. They decided to take the cast off and do more serious testing to see what was the real cause of the problem. In June, five months after her skiing accident, the doctor gave tragic news to Montse's dad: What she had was a tumor in her leg, and it was cancerous. The cancer had already spread, and there was not much they could do to save her life. They could try radiation treatments, but the cancer was irreversible. Montse's mom and dad took the news with so much peace and surrender to God's will. They decided to not tell Montse the seriousness of her condition at this time.

Montse started radiation treatments right away, in the hopes of shrinking the tumor; She had to go to the hospital every day for a month. Her family did not own a car, so Montse and her mom would have to wait for a taxi to come down the street to take them to the hospital. Sometimes the waits for a taxi were very long, and Montse was in a lot of pain standing, but always offering to Jesus all her difficulties. On a few occasions, Montse and her mother ended up walking to the hospital, after no taxis showed up!.

Montse started to wonder what her illness was, since the pain only got worse, and it was getting hard to walk. "Well, Mom, are you going to tell me what I've got?" Monste asked her mother one late night. Her mom and dad had been praying to discern if it was time to tell Montse about her illness. So, Montse's parents decided not to delay it any further: "Montse, you have cancer." She was startled for a second and asked: "Couldn't they cut my leg off?" Her dad explained to her that the doctors had considered everything and that the possibility of cutting her leg off was out. Montse left her parent's room, and went into her own room, where she knelt down by the image of the Blessed

Mother and began to pray. She told Jesus "Whatever you want, Jesus". Then she sat down to do her nightly examination of conscience and prayed three Hail Mary's and she got into her bed. When her mom came to check on her, she was already sleeping. Montse had taken the news with courage, peace and serenity.

From then on, Montse spoke of her illness with naturalness and humility, never wanting to be the center of attention, or the center of special treatments. She knew that she only had a few months to live, and decided to live them as best she could, continuing her studies, family life, going out with her friends, etc., but most of all her plan of life, which she kept with a lot of care. She decided to identify herself with Jesus on the Cross by being "heroic" in the little things of each day, especially in dealing with excruciating pain all the time, without complaining, without letting anyone know that she was hurting. She had the ability to endure her illness, without attracting attention to herself.

After Christmas time, her cancer progressed rapidly. It was during this stage of her sickness that she lived so closed to God, that externally a person couldn't notice that she was in pain. Her leg continued to swell and the pain became unbearable, which made it impossible for her to sleep at night. Her leg got so swollen that the skin tore open and they had to cover it with bandages, which were necessary to remove every day to clean the wound. Montse accepted these treatments cheerfully and was very thankful to those who took care of her. She started to loose her appetite, and eating became very difficult to her, but she offered up every bite for different intentions, in particular for the Pope.

On Holy Thursday, 1959, Montse received the anointing of the sick. While praying the Holy Rosary, surrounded by her family and friends, Monste died peacefully. Her life had been simple and short, but so full of the love of God. Her cause of canonization was opened in 1962.

LaVergne, TN USA
03 November 2009
162658LV00001B